Printed in the US
Published by Harrod Publishing LLC
Photos GoogleImages.com

H.O.P.E Helping Other People Excel

ISBN: 9798575444466

                    H.O.P.E.

The Purpose

This booklet offers clear guidance and support for people starting dialysis for the first time. I want to share my personal experiences and lessons learned because they can help and comfort others facing similar challenges.

Throughout my journey, I have faced many challenges and successes that helped me understand what it means to live with dialysis. I want to share my experiences to explain this treatment's emotional and practical sides. I will cover everything from preparing for the first appointment to learning about different types of dialysis and handling potential side effects. I hope my stories will guide others on this path.

Additionally, I will offer some practical advice on navigating the changes in daily life that dialysis may bring, including dietary adjustments, scheduling treatments, and finding your support.

This booklet aims to provide you with encouragement and tips to help ease your transition into this new phase of life, making the journey feel less daunting and more manageable.

H.O.P.E. Dedication

This book is dedicated to the courageous men and women who embark on the challenging journey of dialysis treatment. Your unwavering resilience and determination in the face of adversity are a profound inspiration to all of us. Each step in navigating this intricate process showcases your strength and fortitude.

I also want to express my gratitude to the dedicated doctors, nurses, and technicians whose expertise and commitment to patient care are indispensable. Their tireless efforts do not go unnoticed, as they provide medical support and emotional encouragement during this difficult time.

A special acknowledgment is warranted for the exceptional staff at DaVita Lakeside in Clinton, Maryland. Their extensive knowledge, genuine compassion, and unwavering support create a nurturing environment that significantly impacts the lives of those undergoing treatment. From the front desk team to the healthcare professionals, every staff member plays a vital role in ensuring patients feel valued and understood.

Your collective efforts are commendable, and this book is a testament to the dialysis community's strength, unity, and resilience. I appreciate your dedication to improving the lives of so many.

LET'S START HERE

I never imagined that I would have to face the reality of dialysis treatment three times a week. It all began when I received the shocking news that my kidneys were not functioning correctly. When the doctor explained my condition, a wave of agitation washed over me. I was overwhelmed with questions and confusion, desperately trying to understand why this was happening to me. My thoughts raced as I grappled with the implications of my diagnosis.

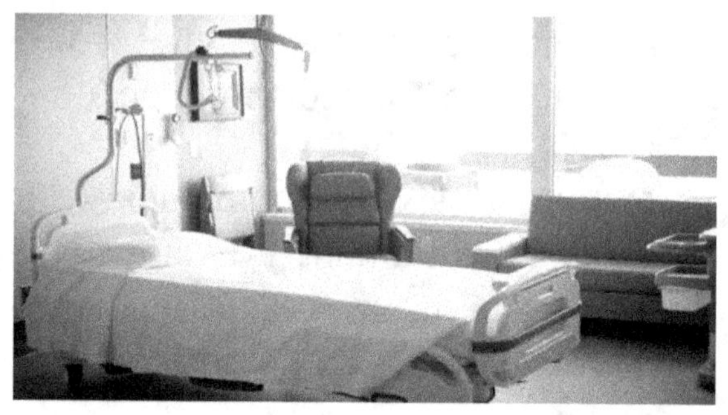

My first encounter with the dialysis process took place in the hospital, where I was introduced to various aspects of the treatment. I watched as medical professionals prepared the dialysis equipment, explaining each step. It was all so overwhelming and surreal as I tried to process the fact that my body was failing in such a critical way.

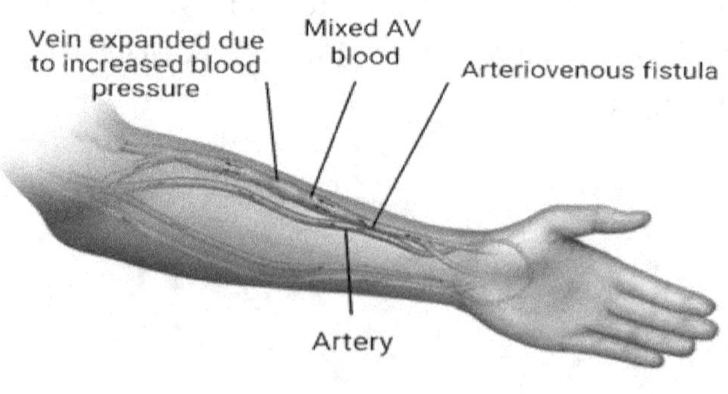

H.O.P.E.

I underwent surgery to have a fistula graft placed in my forearm. This procedure was necessary to facilitate my outpatient treatment for kidney dialysis. The surgery involved creating a durable connection between my blood vessels, allowing efficient access to my bloodstream. After the operation, I was instructed on how to care for the graft as I transitioned to outpatient therapy and began my journey toward recovery.

When I embarked on my outpatient treatment at DaVita Lakeside Dialysis, I found myself immersed in a whirlwind of emotional struggle. The prospect of adjusting my daily life to accommodate these critical sessions loomed over me like a dark cloud. Each time I stepped through the doors of DaVita Lakeside, a wave of apprehension washed over me, accompanied by a deep-seated reluctance to confront this new reality. The environment was both familiar and foreign, filled with the quiet hum of machines and the soft murmur of conversations—each visit served as a poignant reminder of the significant lifestyle changes I was compelled to make.

H.O.P.E.

Despite the initial weight of my feelings, I must take a moment to shed light on the remarkable technicians at

DaVita.

Their unwavering professionalism, paired with a genuine sense of compassion, transformed what could have been a daunting ordeal into a more manageable experience. They approached each session with warmth and understanding, making my time there feel less like a burden and more like a collaborative journey toward my well-being. With their support, the process became not just bearable but also a pathway of encouragement and connection in the midst of the challenges I faced.

I came to the important realization that I had to confront my own behavior because my attitude had become a major obstacle in my life. I often remind myself of the saying, "Your attitude determines your altitude," and it was becoming increasingly evident that I wasn't making any progress or reaching new heights where I was. I felt stuck and frustrated, and it was clear that a change was necessary. I needed to reassess my mindset and make a conscious effort to improve my outlook, as I understood that my future success depended on it.

I took the initiative to educate myself about the treatment options available to me thoroughly. By researching and understanding the various methods, potential benefits,

and side effects, I gained a clearer perspective. This knowledge empowered me and made me feel more comfortable and accepting of the entire process. As a result, I was better equipped to navigate my journey with confidence and a positive mindset.

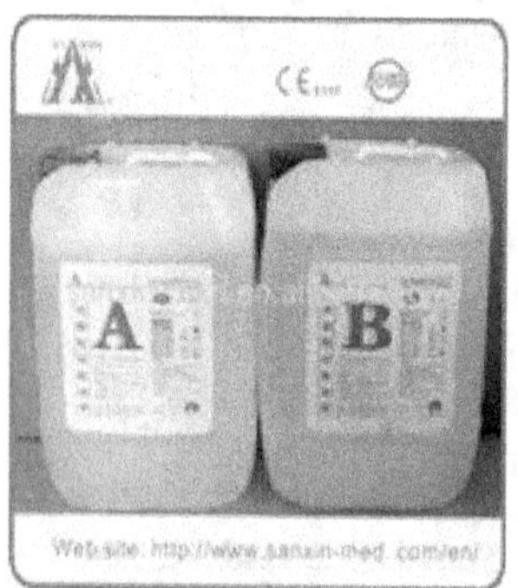

Patients who have severe problems with their kidneys need a dialysis machine to remove harmful substances from their blood. The dialysis machine has one area containing the patient's blood and another location.

These two areas are separated by a Semipermeable membrane through which small molecules can diffuse. Small waste products such as Urea Defuse from the flood into the Dialysate. The Dialysate that flows out of the machine is then discarded.

In the Hemodialysis machine, where the filtering takes place, blood containing waste flows into the machine from the patient's body. Used Dialysate carries waste out of the Machine and is discarded. A Semipermeable Membrane keeps the blood and Dialysate from mixing but allows waste to pass. Waste from the blood diffuses through the membrane and into the Dialysate. Clean blood is then returned to the patient's body.

Excerpt from P.T.S. from Life Sciences Learning Center. Copyright 2009 University of Rochester

LET ME SHARE A TRUE STORY WITH YOU

There was a gentleman who often sat directly across from me in the treatment center. He frequently voiced his dissatisfaction with being in treatment, expressing frustration and annoyance almost every day. His complaints seemed to overshadow any positive aspects of the experience.

One day, after he had finished yet another round of grievances — lamenting the monotony of the days and the program's challenges — I decided to interject. I waited patiently for him to finish, and then I said, "You're still alive."

He paused, taken aback by my words. There was a moment of silence as he processed what I had said. Finally, he looked at me and replied, "You are so right!"

It struck me how often he focused on the negative, to the point where he had lost sight of the most vital truth: he was still alive and could change his circumstances. That realization resonated with him and highlighted how easily we can overlook the positives during our struggles.

After that initial period, we developed a friendship. A technician who had known the gentleman for some time shared with me that he had made significant positive changes in his life. It was encouraging to hear how he had turned things around after overcoming some personal challenges with his attitude.

Remarkably, after improving his outlook and mindset, he was able to receive a kidney transplant, which was a crucial turning point in his health journey. I felt a deep sense of satisfaction knowing that I had contributed, even in a small way, to his change in perspective.

Then he returned to visit me, and I was thrilled to see him. He looked good and full of life, strikingly contrasting his appearance during our last meeting. His transformation was remarkable; his energy was palpable, and he carried an inspiring air of confidence. It was heartwarming to witness the physical changes—his healthier complexion and fitter physique—and the emotional growth he had experienced. We spent hours catching up, sharing stories and laughter, and seeing his progress on his journey filled me with joy. His positivity and determination resonated deeply with me, and I felt fortunate to be a part of this moment.

In Life we often complained about situations, but instead of complaining, we should take that energy to get answers for our situation.

H.O.P.E.

Every person's journey through life is distinct and filled with individual experiences. I would love to take a moment to share my journey, highlighting the challenges I've faced, the lessons I've learned, and the growth I've experienced along the way.

In life, we will have necessary interruptions. One question I asked myself is, DO YOU WANT TO LIVE?   You must get your mind right when confronted with treatment decisions.   And you know the answers that keep coming up: YES, I WANT TO LIVE!

> If your kidneys fail, dialysis can save your life. Dialysis is not just a medical treatment; it can also affect every aspect of your life. You must get your mind right for the journey.

If your kidneys fail, undergoing dialysis can be crucial for your survival.

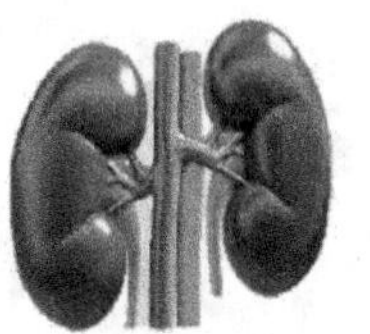Dialysis is a medical treatment that artificially removes waste products and excess fluid from the blood, functioning as a substitute for the natural filtering process of healthy kidneys. Beyond its life-saving capabilities, dialysis can significantly influence various aspects of your daily life and overall well-being. It may affect your routine, dietary choices, emotional health, and support network, making understanding this treatment's medical and lifestyle implications essential. Taking charge of your health journey with this knowledge can help you navigate the challenges that come along with kidney failure and dialysis.

Going through the complexities of treatment options can feel daunting and overwhelming for many individuals. Life is full of inevitable interruptions, and these challenges can complicate our decision-making processes. When I find myself at a crossroads regarding treatment, I take a moment to reflect deeply on my priorities. I ask myself the fundamental question: do I genuinely want to live, and what kind of life do I envision for myself? This introspection helps clarify my values and guides my decisions, allowing me to approach treatment purposefully.

And you know the answer keeps coming up: YES! That's why it's so important to get as much information as possible.

As I continue with my treatment journey, I've come to realize that my experiences can vary significantly from day to day. Some days, I feel energized and hopeful, while others can be more challenging and draining. Regardless of these ups and downs, I firmly believe in maintaining a positive attitude throughout the process.

One particular day, I spoke with a gentleman expressing his frustrations and complaints about his situation. With gratitude in my heart, I reminded him that we are still alive and should be thankful for that!

Focusing on a better outcome is most important, even in difficult times.

It's important to recognize that when our bodies experience changes or discomfort, it's crucial to communicate these concerns with someone we trust. For those who are married, sharing these experiences with a spouse can provide emotional support and reassurance. They can also encourage us to seek medical advice if necessary. Additionally, consulting with a healthcare professional is vital, as they have the knowledge and expertise to assess our symptoms accurately. Early detection of potential health issues can significantly affect treatment outcomes.

Identifying a problem early on can be life-saving, highlighting the importance of open dialogue about our health with those closest to us and medical professionals.

During my travels across various states, I have been incredibly fortunate to discover that *DaVita* treatment centers are easily accessible in so many locations. Each center provides high-quality care and support for individuals undergoing dialysis, making it convenient for patients to receive the treatment they need, regardless of where they are. It's reassuring to know that these facilities are widespread, ensuring that essential health services are available to those who require them.

Before the pandemic, I sought treatment in several states, each offering unique experiences and settings. In San Diego, California, I appreciated the sunny atmosphere and the proximity to the beautiful beaches, which provided a sense of calm during my visits. North Carolina also played a significant role in my treatment journey, with its serene landscapes charming, welcoming, and peaceful.

Ocean City, Maryland, was another location where I received care, and I loved the vibrant seaside environment and the bustling boardwalk, which lifted my spirits during my time there. However, my favorite place for treatment has to be Clinton, Maryland. The warm community atmosphere and the care I received made it a truly special experience. Each location contributed to my healing journey differently, but Clinton holds a special place in my heart.

SOME KEYS I'VE APPLIED TO MY JOURNEY

EDUCATE YOURSELF: Get as much information as you can. Anyone on this journey will find there is much information out there. Read, Ask Questions, Read, Ask Questions, Read, Ask Questions. Keep educating yourself about what you are going through. Keep good communication with your doctors.

DON'T SETTLE FOR THE FIRST DIAGNOSES

Be informed and know what you are taking; ask about the risks versus benefits of each new drug you start. Make informed decisions about your care, as there are many choices today. If you start the discussion with your doctors, you can allow them to collaborate, which is to your benefit.

BE YOUR OWN ADVOCATE

This is important to getting what you need. If this is too much for you to handle alone, ask someone to walk you through this process. Sometimes hearing the news, we don't always hear. Having another set of ears will help when your emotions have settled; they can give you what was said.

Keeping good notes is imperative regarding dosage, Albumin, Hemoglobin, Calcium Levels, Blood Pressure, Phosphorus Levels, PTH Intact, Potassium, spKdt/V Dialysis, Fluid Weight Gain, and H.G.B./1c (gLYCOHGb) in between appointments on what is going on throughout your body.

KEEP LEARNING

You have to know what will give you the most healing. Keep thinking and learning.

TO YOURSELF AND OTHERS - BE KIND

While you are your best advocate, invite someone to walk with you on your journey: a walking partner or shopping partner. Allow yourself to rest after treatments and spend time with loved ones. This is good medicine. Listen to your body. Make time for what brings you peace, heal, and allow yourself to receive.

YOUR DIET IS IMPORTANT

You may not be able to eat those three big meals we are used to eating. The suggestion is six small meals every three hours. Eat thoughtfully, and you will feel the difference. There are many values to know in renal disease, and adjust your diet accordingly. Be informed.

ORGANIZE YOUR TRAVELS

In organizing your travels, plan ahead. When I've traveled out of town, I had to first communicate with DaVita, and they informed me of the DaVita Center in the state where I would be traveling. Another lesson I've learned is to take control of where I can. Take steps to manage your health, organize your surroundings, and stay positive—*you are not a victim*. Keep a list of questions as they arise to be ready the next time you talk with your health professional.

Filing or keeping track of your labs and medications as they change helps you look back on them and often helps to look at the whole story. If you are missing exercise, make a plan that suits you. It makes us feel weak when things seemingly spiral out of our control—do something! Join a support group, and see how you may be able to help others—there is strength in numbers for sure! The more I can control, the less that is beyond me, and the more gratitude I feel for what is going well. Look at the positive and do what you can to see the good in each situation. With chronic illness, some days, this is tough! Realize it, feel it, and then ask yourself if you can do more to help meet your goals. Sometimes, there is not much more we can do than practice gratitude.

LEAN ON YOUR SUPPORT

They are within reach. All you have to do is ask. When making a significant decision, it will be helpful to have a friend to talk things over with. I feel blessed with great support, but one person who is very helpful in this part of my journey is my wife. She has been there through some of the rough times, emergency room visits, and hospital stays, and she continuously checks on me while I'm in treatment. She has been there through the highs and lows—know we will have them.

> In the process, you must know your role because it's not only the doctors, but there is an important part you play in your treatment!
>
> Ask yourself

KNOW WHEN TO PROCEED

Take as much time as you need to gather what you need for this journey. Everyone is different, so the process will have slight variations. Once you focus on your healing, all decisions will point to that. The decision to move forward will give you added strength and confidence. You must stay positive and enjoy your life. I have found wisdom to be one of my critical elements.

This is not an accident.
I am ALIVE because there's more to my life!

I had been on dialysis for 4.5 years. During the final process, I should review my medical history, physical examination, and psychological evaluation, meet with financial counselors, and consult various specialists to determine my best options. It would be best to meet the criteria and then wait for your opportunity. Surround yourself with a positive support system.

Encouragement is GOOD Medicine!

DON'T YOU LOSE HOPE!

Prayer

Heavenly Father, thank You for your new life. Thank you for forgiving me of all my sins. It makes me brand new. I believe Jesus died for me and rose again so I can live for You. Fill me with Your spirit so I can know, serve, and follow You for the rest of my life. My life is not my own, so I give it to You today. Thank You for a new life. In Jesus' name, I pray, AMEN.

THE OTHER SIDE OF HOPE

(def: a feeling of expectation and a desire for a sure thing to happen)

The book I wrote previously, H.O.P.E., was a great accomplishment for me. As I started this new chapter of my life after having the kidney transplant, I had no idea whatsoever that these events would happen the way that they did.

Let's go back to Friday, February 19, 2021, when I had dialysis at the DaVita Lakeside Dialysis Center.

I had come for my treatment as I usually did for the days that I was scheduled. One of the technicians said to me that they hoped that I would get a kidney that weekend. That was very nice for them for the words of encouragement.

Well, my primary Dr. Chike Onwuka, had told me some weeks earlier that I would be receiving a kidney within ninety days. Now, I was already on the top of the kidney transplant list at The Johns Hopkins Hospital in

Baltimore, Maryland. I was also testing to get on Georgetown Hospital's list and was currently going through a series of tests so I could be placed on their list as well. I later received news stating that, as of December 2020, there would be no advantage to being on multiple lists.

That's why I was trying to be on Georgetown Hospital's list. I thought I was no longer on the Johns Hopkins Hospital list because of the new rules. I had been going to the DaVita clinic for five years, and it seemed like nothing was happening well. The people were great! I was referring to donors. My outlook was still that I was trusting God through this process.

We must learn to be patient because things won't always happen when we want them to.

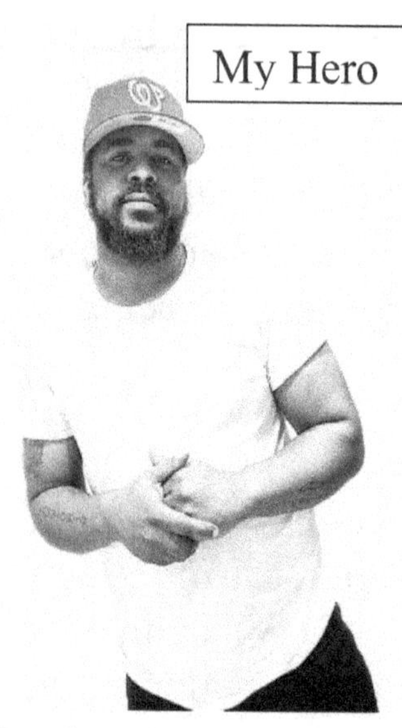

Our friend Alicia Walker comes with bad news about her son Curtis. Curtis had a head injury and had to be rushed to The Johns Hopkins Hospital. When he arrived at the hospital, they conducted a series of tests to determine if there was any brain activity. During the last round of tests, he unfortunately did not survive. Any mother would find it incredibly difficult to endure such a situation. Despite her grief, she expressed a desire for me to be one of her son's recipients of his kidneys.

The medical team at Johns Hopkins Hospital reached out to me with an urgent offer: they had a kidney available for transplant, and they wanted to know if I was interested in accepting it. I felt overwhelmed as the news came in; everything was happening so quickly that I needed a moment to gather my thoughts. After being on dialysis for five long years, the prospect of a kidney transplant was both exciting and intimidating.

I decided to ask the nurse if they could call me back later so I could process the information without feeling rushed. This decision was not just about me; it would significantly impact my life and family. I turned to my wife to discuss how she felt about the situation. After explaining how quickly things were moving, I looked to her for guidance. She responded with enthusiasm, saying, "What? You better take that kidney! This is a great opportunity! Let's do this!" Her support gave me the confidence to move forward with the decision.

I carefully packed a bag with all the essentials, ensuring I had everything I might need, and then we set off for the hospital. As we approached the impressive facade of Johns Hopkins Hospital, a sense of nervous anticipation overcame me. This was no ordinary place; it was a legendary institution known for its cutting-edge medical breakthroughs and exceptional patient care. I had heard stories about how doctors from all corners of the globe came here, drawn by the opportunity to collaborate and learn from the best in their fields. Standing there, I couldn't help but feel excitement and apprehension as I prepared to step inside such an esteemed place.

On March 20, 2021, I made my way to Johns Hopkins University for a visit. When I arrived, the staff welcomed me warmly and guided me to my room. To my delight, the room offered a spectacular view of Baltimore. I could see the bustling cityscape, with its iconic landmarks and vibrant streets, which made my stay even more enjoyable. The experience was enriching and memorable, and I couldn't help but feel excitement about the time I was about to spend there.

On that Saturday morning, the atmosphere in the hospital was tense yet hopeful, as a significant surgery was scheduled for that day. However, just hours before the procedure began, unexpected complications arose in the operating room. Medical staff encountered a few logistical issues that threatened to delay the surgery, causing concern among the team and the patient's family. The nurses rushed to address the problems while the surgeons discussed possible solutions to ensure they could proceed as planned.

I had the entire day to settle in, and the excitement was overwhelming; I could hardly rest. Although I experienced mixed emotions, I was finally there. I remember my wife, LaWanna, and my grandson, Connor, waiting in the room with me. I was so glad they were by my side.

The doctors entered my hospital room, bringing a sense of professionalism and reassurance with them. They carefully explained the treatment plan they had developed, outlining each step of the procedure ahead of me. As I absorbed their words, a wave of calm washed over me, easing the anxiety inside.

Sitting in that sterile environment, my mind wandered back to simpler times when I enjoyed good health. I couldn't help but reflect on the journey that had led me to this point, filled with moments of uncertainty and fear. Yet, despite everything, I had reached this crucial juncture, and it felt like more than mere chance; it seemed like a divine appointment orchestrated by /a higher power.

I am deeply grateful to the Walker family for their kindness and support. Their willingness to help had made all the difference in my situation.

On that significant Sunday, March 21, 2021, at around 8:30 a.m., I was wheeled down to the operating room, the chill of the hallway contrasting with the warmth of their compassion. The doctors who greeted me in the OR took the time to review the procedure again, ensuring that I felt informed and ready.

They reassured me that my blood and kidney types were a perfect match, a crucial detail that brought me hope amidst the uncertainty. Their dedication and expertise made me feel safe and supported as I prepared for the operation.

When I regained consciousness, I found myself in the recovery room, surrounded by the reassuring beeping of monitors and the soft murmur of medical staff. A nurse smiled at me and explained that everything had gone successfully. Filled with relief, I reached for my phone and called my wife. When I heard her voice on the other end, I could feel her joy and excitement through the line, even though she was shocked to discover I had the strength to speak. My heart swelled with gratitude as I thought about how lucky I am to have LaWanna by my side; she has been my rock throughout this journey.

THE HEALING PROCESS BEGINS NOW!

A few days after the surgery, I made it a point to get up and walk around my home to help regain my strength. Each morning, I would carefully rise from my bed, ensuring I felt steady on my feet. I started with short walks, gradually increasing my distance as I felt more comfortable. On some days, I could walk around my hospital floor three times, feeling a sense of accomplishment with each lap I completed. Each step was a small victory on my journey to recovery.

The staff at Johns Hopkins Hospital was incredible! Various doctors explained clearly all the vital medications I would need to take.

The wealth of information I received was undeniably extensive, yet it sometimes felt overwhelming. It became clear that the first change I needed was within my mindset. To truly embark on a path to recovery, I had to learn to embrace certain truths and experiences that, while daunting, were crucial for my progress.

Encouraged by the doctors' consistently positive reports, I discovered a renewed determination within myself, motivating me to strive even harder on my healing journey.

On March 28th, I finally returned home, and a wave of relief washed over me as I stepped through the door. My wife had gone above and beyond to create a welcoming atmosphere, carefully preparing our home to support my recovery. To assist me during this transition, I arranged for nurses to visit regularly, providing guidance and help as I adjusted to my new routine.

For now, I found myself confined to the first floor of my home, fully aware that climbing the stairs was too risky as my body healed from the kidney transplant surgery. The faint scent of antiseptics lingered in the air, constantly reminding me of my recent struggles. Despite these limitations, I was fiercely determined to regain strength and independence.

Each day, I stepped forward with a sense of purpose, my feet firmly planted on the path toward recovery. The encouraging words of my doctors echoed in my mind, serving as a guiding light as I navigated the challenges ahead. I consciously tried to pace myself, aware that patience was crucial. With each moment that passed, I could feel a quiet transformation within me—a gradual yet undeniable improvement pulsing through my body. Despite the flicker of hope in my heart, I clung to a sense of caution, fully aware that every small victory was a vital building block on my journey to full recovery.

After navigating the constant whirlwind of daily life, I finally found a moment to pause and breathe. The world around me quieted, and I felt the weight of stress lifting from my shoulders, allowing my mind to settle into a calm state. This was my opportunity to reflect deeply on my experiences and to gather my thoughts about the next steps in my recovery journey. It was a sacred time for introspection and healing, and I felt a profound readiness to embrace this transformative process. The air was filled with possibilities, and I was prepared to explore the depths of my mind and spirit, nurturing the seeds of growth and renewal.

I have finally reached a point in my recovery where I no longer need the nurses' assistance. This milestone is bittersweet for me; I feel a sense of pride in my newfound independence, yet I remain grateful for the invaluable lessons they taught me. They instructed me on essential aspects of self-care, including managing my medication and recognizing the signs my body needs. Their support was crucial during my journey, and I genuinely appreciate all the guidance they provided during my time of need.

I began making gradual changes and taking steps to progress in my healing journey. When my doctor finally cleared me to drive again, I felt a wave of joy and freedom—it was as if I had been liberated from a long period of restriction. The recovery experience has been a rollercoaster; some days are filled with positivity and hope, while others present challenges and setbacks. I've realized that experiencing both the highs and lows is essential to my journey back to normalcy.

To stay on track with my recovery journey, I have dedicated myself to the daily practice of monitoring my vital signs and glucose levels. This routine has emerged as a critical component of my self-care regimen, empowering me to take proactive steps in overseeing my health. Each morning and evening, I carefully check these essential indicators, which allows me to stay informed about my body's condition and make any necessary adjustments to my lifestyle or treatment. By understanding the importance of these measurements, I cultivate a more profound sense of control and awareness, guiding me toward healing and well-being.

It has now been over three years since I underwent my kidney transplant surgery, a life-changing procedure that marked the beginning of a new chapter in my health journey. Looking back, I can still remember the emotions I felt on that day, filled with hope and anxiety as I prepared for the operation that would give me a second chance at life. I Am Grateful!

As 2024 draws to a close, I find myself standing at the threshold of 2025, brimming with anticipation and new ambitions. With a fresh sense of purpose, I am ready to explore uncharted territories. My faith in God serves as a guiding light, and the unwavering support from my wife reinforces my courage to face the challenges ahead. I am acutely aware that there are still lessons to be learned—insights that will bolster my hope and resilience as I navigate the journey toward a brighter future on the other side.

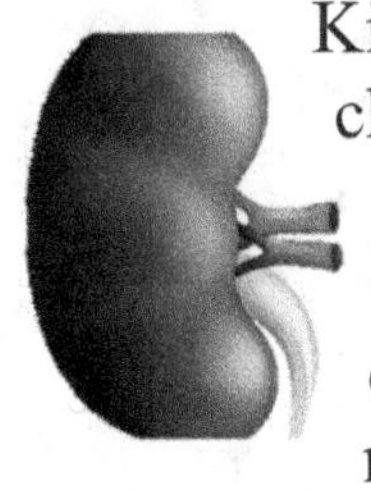 Kidney disease symptoms include changes in urination, swelling, and fatigue. Kidney disease is sometimes called a "silent disease" because it can have few or no symptoms.

Urination changes

Urinating more or less frequently

Urinating more at night

Urine that is foamy, bubbly, darker, paler, or bloody

Difficulty urinating

Pain or burning when urinating

Swelling

Swelling in the ankles, feet, hands, or face

Puffiness around the legs and ankles

Fatigue, tiredness, inability to concentrate, and generally unwell feeling.

H . O . P . E .

Other symptoms:

Weight loss or poor appetite

Shortness of breath

Itchy skin

Back pain

High blood pressure

Nausea and vomiting

Bad breath and a metallic taste in the mouth

If you have persistent symptoms of kidney disease, you should see a doctor.

Symptoms

-Chronic kidney disease

Contents

Overview

Symptoms

Diagnosis

Treatment

Living with

Prevention

Many people with chronic kidney disease (CKD) will not have symptoms because it does not usually cause problems until it reaches an advanced stage.

Early stages of CKD

Kidney disease does not tend to cause symptoms at an early stage.

This is because the body can usually cope with significantly reduced kidney function.

Kidney disease is often only diagnosed at this stage if a routine test for another condition, such as a blood or urine test, detects a possible problem.

If it's found at an early stage, medicine and regular tests to monitor it may help prevent its progression.

Later stages of CKD

Some symptoms can develop if kidney disease is not found early or it gets worse despite treatment.

Symptoms can include:

weight loss and poor appetite

swollen ankles, feet, or hands – as a result of water retention (oedema)

shortness of breath

tiredness

blood in your pee (urine)

an increased need to pee – particularly at night

difficulty sleeping (insomnia)

itchy skin

muscle cramps

feeling sick

headaches

erectile dysfunction in men

This stage of CKD is known as kidney failure, end-stage renal disease, or established renal failure. It may eventually require treatment with dialysis or a kidney transplant.

When to get medical advice

See a GP if you have persistent or worrying symptoms that you think could be caused by kidney disease.

Many less severe conditions can cause the symptoms of kidney disease, so it's crucial to get a proper diagnosis.

If you do have CKD, it's best to get it diagnosed as soon as possible. Kidney disease can be diagnosed by having blood and urine tests.

Kidney patients often refer to their disease progression using stages, which can be confusing to those new to kidney disease.

In an ideal world, renal patients would be diagnosed at birth or immediately after the onset of specific symptoms. Unfortunately, this is not the case. Many patients, particularly Alport syndrome patients, are diagnosed long after their kidney function has started to decline.

To make matters worse, one in every three American adults is at risk for kidney disease. To categorize the renal function of the 26 million American adults with chronic kidney disease, the National Kidney Foundation (NKF) created a five-stage guideline. Read on to learn more about testing, early detection, and the stages of kidney disease.

Testing and Early Detection

Many people are unaware renal disease can lack noticeable symptoms until it is too late. Therefore, testing is crucial, especially if you are a high-risk patient. NKF offers <u>free urine testing</u> for high-risk patients. The Alport Syndrome Foundation strongly encourages anyone with a family history of the disease to be tested immediately and regularly. A simple urine test can determine the amount of protein your body expels, while a blood draw can determine how well your kidneys filter and remove waste. The results of these quick tests can immeasurably impact your future health.

Patients with Alport syndrome should have regular kidney screenings, but even family members who don't have Alport syndrome can be at risk of developing kidney disease from other causes. Absolutely anyone over the age of 60 is advised to be tested, as are those with high blood pressure, a BMI (body mass index) over 30, and/or diabetes. According to NKF, African Americans, Hispanics, Asians, Pacific Islanders, and American Indians also have a greater risk of renal disease. Early detection of renal disease provides greater flexibility in treatment options, may prolong the time before dialysis, and can allow you to make daily life changes, helping to maintain current/remaining renal function.

While some patients experience little or no visible symptoms, it is important to recognize the potential warning signs of renal disease. These include, but are not limited to, overall malaise, poor appetite, lack of focus/concentration, nocturnal muscle cramping, sleep irritability, and swollen feet/ankles. If initial testing indicates kidney disease, subsequent testing may occur, including more bloodwork, kidney ultrasound, or a biopsy.

Once it is established you have kidney disease, your doctor will measure how well your kidneys filter blood using a test called a Glomerular Filtration Rate (GFR). The resulting GFR will determine your particular stage on a scale of 1-5. Generally speaking, outward symptoms are experienced only during and after stage 3, though some exceptions exist.

Five Stages of Kidney Disease
Alport Syndrome

alportsyndrome.org

Symptoms and Treatment Options

Stages 1-2:

Unnoticeable external symptoms.

- Diet changes include limiting sodium and protein intake.
- Ingestion of fruits, veggies, and whole grains is advised.
- Control of cholesterol, blood sugar, and blood pressure.
- Exercise/staying active is recommended.
- No smoking.
- Regular Checkups to monitor GFR.
- Medication such as ACE (angiotensin-converting enzyme) inhibitors and ARBs (angiotensin receptor blockers) are prescribed to help slow renal decline.

H.O.P.E.

* Please note: For Alport patients, starting an ACE is <u>recommended</u> not at a certain stage of kidney function or GFR but when the urine protein to creatinine ratio is above 0.2 as measured in a simple urinalysis test. Regular measurement of urine protein levels is recommended beginning at one year of age in children with Alport syndrome and at least annually for all patients of all ages.

Stage 3:

At this stage, symptoms of kidney disease are very apparent. These include fluid retention, changes in urine color, kidney pain, and extreme fatigue.

- Finding a nephrologist is essential at this stage. A dietician is also normally recommended.
- Phosphorous and calcium consumption will be limited in your daily diet.
- Maintaining all the treatment recommendations from stages 1-2 is crucial.

- Medication such as ACE (angiotensin-converting enzyme) inhibitors and ARBs (angiotensin receptor blockers) are prescribed to help slow renal decline.*

* Please note: For individuals diagnosed with Alport syndrome, initiating treatment with an angiotensin-converting enzyme (ACE) inhibitor is advisable when the urine protein-to-creatinine ratio surpasses 0.2. Routine urinalysis, a straightforward and non-invasive test, can determine this threshold. It is important to recognize that the timing for beginning ACE therapy depends not solely on the patient's kidney function or glomerular filtration rate (GFR), but rather on the presence of significant proteinuria, as indicated by the urine test results.

In addition, regular monitoring of urine protein levels is crucial for all patients with Alport syndrome, regardless of age. This should be conducted at least annually to effectively track any changes in proteinuria and assess the progression of the disease. Monitoring helps adjust treatment plans and ensure timely interventions to preserve kidney function and overall health.

Stage 4:

In addition to the symptoms of renal disease listed in the previous stages, patients can experience a foul, metallic taste in their mouth and bad breath due to excess urea in the blood.

- At this stage, dialysis and/or renal transplantation are likely in the near future. Your nephrologist will review the types of dialysis with you in preparation,
- Patients may become anemic during stage 4 as their red blood cell count drops.

Stage 5

Loss of appetite and limited urine output are common during this stage.

- The only treatments for stage 5 are hemodialysis, peritoneal dialysis, or kidney transplantation.
- Potassium intake is closely monitored.

- Vitamins are often prescribed.

What foods are bad for the kidneys?
Renal diet

Foods to avoid

Other foods

Summary

People with kidney disease typically need to follow a diet low in sodium, protein, potassium, and phosphorus. This means limiting or avoiding foods such as avocados, brown rice, and chips.

The kidneys perform many crucial functions and are a Trusted Source for Health. They filter waste products and excess fluid from the body and remove them through urine. They also regulate the body's mineral balance and produce a hormone that stimulates red blood cell production.

Waste products can build up in a person's blood when they have kidney disease. A doctor may recommend dietary changes to help manage the condition and support kidney function.

This article explains which foods people with kidney disease should avoid or limit and provides an overview of the renal (or "kidney-friendly") diet.

Renal diet

A specialist kidney dietitian will typically work with people with kidney disease to tailor a diet to their needs.

A kidney-friendly diet, also called a renal diet, may vary slightly depending on the stage of a person's kidney disease.

For example, those in the early stages of chronic kidney disease (CKD) should limit their sodium and possibly protein intake.

In the later stages Trusted Source of CKD, known as kidney failure, an individual should follow a diet that limits sodium, potassium, and phosphorus.

Learn about the link between kidney disease and potassium.

Foods to avoid

A dietitian may ask that individuals following a renal diet avoid the following foods:

1. Canned foods

Sodium, a main ingredient in salt, is a natural mineral often found in large quantities in canned foods. Manufacturers typically add Trusted Source sodium to canned items to increase shelf life and enhance taste.

With CKD, the kidneys cannot eliminate excess sodium as they should. This means people with CKD should avoid or limit eating canned goods such as soup, vegetables, and beans.

Choosing canned foods labeled "low sodium" and draining the contents can help reduce the amount of sodium a person consumes.

2. Whole wheat bread

A buildup of phosphorus and potassium can cause problems for people with CKD. Because whole wheat bread contains high amounts of these minerals, people with CKD should instead choose white bread.

For example, one slice of whole wheat bread contains 76.3 mg Trusted Source of phosphorus and 90 mg of potassium. White bread, on the other hand, contains 31.6 mg Trusted Source of phosphorus and 32.8 mg of potassium.

If a person does not wish to stop eating whole wheat bread entirely, they could instead consider reducing the amount they eat. For example, they could eat just one slice with a meal rather than two.

3. Dark-colored drinks

Many manufacturers of dark-colored drinks add phosphorus to enhance flavor, prolong shelf life, and prevent discoloration.

Phosphorus in its additive form, found in dark cola and beer, is highly absorbable by the human body and is not a recommended Source for those following a renal diet.

However, root beer is an exception to this as it contains no phosphorus Trusted Source.

4. Avocados

While healthcare professionals generally consider avocados a beneficial addition to a person's diet, people with renal problems may wish to avoid or limit them.

This is because they are high in potassium, with one avocado weighing around 200 g containing 975 mgTrusted Source of potassium. According to the National Kidney Foundation, anything that exceeds 200 mg of potassium per serving is high in potassium.

If needed, a person can still include avocados in their diet, but they should drastically reduce their portion size.

5. Bananas

A large banana contains 487 mg Trusted Source of potassium, meaning a person with CKD should avoid or limit eating this fruit. Many other tropical fruits also have high potassium content.

Pineapples may be a suitable alternative as they contain a much smaller amount Trusted Source of potassium than other tropical fruits.

6. Oranges and orange juice

Oranges and orange juice are a potassium-rich food and drink.

A small orange contains 174mg of potassium, while 250g of Trusted Source orange juice contains as much as 441 mg of potassium.

Alternative fruits that are lower in potassium include grapes, apples, and cranberries.

7. Dried fruits

Dried fruits are concentrated sources of many nutrients found in fresh fruits. This means it can be easier to exceed their recommended daily intake.

People following a renal diet should avoid apricots, dates, prunes, and raisins, all of which are high in potassium.

8. Tomatoes

Tomatoes are another high-potassium fruit that a person following a renal diet should limit.

For reference, a cup (245 g) of tomato sauce contains 728mg of Trusted Source of potassium.

9. Brown rice

While it is nutritious, brown rice has a more Trusted Source of phosphorus and potassium content than white rice.

A cup (155 g) of cooked brown rice contains 149 trusted Sources of phosphorus and 94.6 mg of potassium, while a cup (186 g) of cooked white rice contains 68.8 trusted Sources of phosphorus and 53.9 mg of potassium.

Bulgur, buckwheat, and couscous are also alternatives to brown rice.

10. Dairy

Despite traditionally being promoted for bone health, consuming too much dairy can be detrimental to bone health for people with CKD. Dairy is a natural source of phosphorus and potassium.

A cup (244 g) of whole milk contains 205mg Trusted Source of phosphorus and 322mg of potassium.

Kidney damage can cause excess phosphorus to build up in the blood (known as hyperphosphatemia). This condition can cause the body to pull calcium from the bones, resulting in thin, weak bones.

People following a renal diet should limit dairy products to avoid this buildup of protein waste in the blood.

Coconut milk may be a favorable substitute for people with CKD based on Trusted Source, its low potassium, sodium, and oxalate content.

11. Processed meats

Processed meats are meats that manufacturers have salted, dried, cured, or canned. Some examples include hot dogs, bacon, and pepperoni. They often contain lots of trusted Source salt to improve their taste and preserve flavor.

If a person regularly eats highly processed foods, keeping their sodium intake to 2,300mg daily (the amount recommended by the National Kidney Foundation) may be difficult.

12. Pickles, olives, and relish

Pickles, processed olives, and relish are all cured or pickled foods.

Manufacturers typically add salt rusted Source to the food during the curing or pickling process.

For reference, five green pickled olives (considered a small serving) equate to almost 10%Trusted Source of the daily recommended amount of sodium.

13. Bran cereals, oatmeal, and granola

Many cereals contain a mixture of potassium, phosphorus, and sodium. A person following a renal diet should avoid all of these.

For example, a 30-trusted Source serving of bran flakes contains 160 mg of potassium, 135 mg of phosphorus, and 162mg of sodium, while a 100-trusted Source serving of granola contains 539mg of potassium.

14. Potatoes

Potatoes, including sweet potatoes, are potassium-rich vegetables.

A medium-sized baked potato contains around 610mg of potassium, and a medium-sized sweet potato contains 542mg of potassium.

Leaching is one way to reduce potatoes' high potassium content. This method involves soaking or boiling potatoes in water before cooking, which, according to older research, reduces the original potassium content by at least 50% Trusted Source.

15. Processed foods

Processed foods include pizza, instant noodles, and convenience meals designed for the microwave. These foods typically contain high levels of salt, sugar, and fat.

As mentioned above, the National Kidney Foundation recommends keeping sodium intake to 2,300 mg per day. This may prove not easy if a person regularly eats highly processed foods.

16. Pretzels, chips, and crackers

Foods such as pretzels, chips, and crackers are typically high in sodium and lacking in nutrients. Chips come from potatoes, which are also high in potassium.

A small bag of potato chips contains around 148mg of True Source of sodium and 336mg of potassium, and 60g of pretzels contains roughly 744 mg of True Source of sodium and 134 mg of potassium.

The portion sizes of these snacks can often lead to greater salt intake than intended.

17. Swiss chard, spinach, and beet greens

Due to their high potassium content, many green, leafy vegetables, such as Swiss chard, spinach, and beet greens, may need to be avoided or limited by people following a renal diet.

For example, a cup of raw Swiss chard contains 136mg of Trusted Source of potassium. As with spinach, this vegetable shrinks when boiled, meaning a person may eat more than they would raw. A person with CKD should consider this as it will, in turn, increase their intake of potassium.

Kidney-friendly foods

Although individuals with CKD must adapt their diet, they can still try many suitable options.

People should choose foods with lower sodium, potassium, and phosphorus levels. These include:

Fruit: Options include apples, cranberries, grapes, pineapple, and strawberries.

Vegetables: Options include cauliflower, lettuce, onions, peppers, and radishes.

Baked goods: Options include pita, tortillas, and sourdough bread.

Protein: Options include beef and chicken.

H.O.P.E.

Carbohydrates: Options include white rice and unsalted popcorn.

Learn about other foods that are good for the kidneys.

Summary

If an individual has CKD, doctors typically recommend reducing their potassium, phosphorus, and sodium intake to help manage the condition. The dietary restrictions depend on the stage of the disease.

Although there is a long list of foods that are best to avoid on a renal diet, there is also a wide range of foods that people can eat without affecting their kidney health.

An individual may work with a renal dietitian to find the most suitable diet for them.

medicalnewstoday.com

The National Kidney Foundation
National Capital Area
(800) 622-9010
www.kidney.org

American Kidney Fund
www.kidneyfund.org

National Kidney Registry
www.kidneyregistery.com

H.O.P.E.